WEiGH
YOUR WORDS
and
THROW AWAY
YOUR SCALE!

The Jewish Woman's Guide
to Losing Weight and Feeling Great

Gloria Davidson and Hope Stanger

Targum Publishers

First published 2016
Copyright © 2016 by Gloria Davidson and Hope Stanger
All rights reserved
ISBN: 978-1-56871-607-7

Published by
TARGUM PUBLISHERS
POB 27515
Jerusalem 91274
editor@targumpublishers.com

Distributed by
Ktav Publishers & Distributors Inc.
527 Empire Blvd.
Brooklyn, NY 11225-3121
Tel: 718-972-5449, 201-963-9524
Fax: 718-972-6307, 201-963-0102
www.ktav.com

Printed in Israel

DEDICATION

This book is dedicated to all the Jewish women who are at the point of exasperation from years of weight loss and weight gain. Whether you are young or old, married or single, have children or do not, are a businesswoman or homemaker, a binge eater or someone struggling with an eating disorder, **WE WANT TO HELP – AND WE CAN!**

"You are no longer alone in your weight-loss journey"

With Love,
Gloria and Hope

THANK YOU FROM GLORIA

To my wonderful husband, MENDY, who has made my life complete and made all my dreams come true. Thank you for making me smile every day and fueling my creative energy to complete this book. I love you.

To my parents, JERRY and RENÉE GROSSFIELD, my deeper-than-describable love and appreciation for your constant love, support and encouragement. I am what I am today because of both of you.

To my children, SHIMSHON and NA'AMA NADEL, DANNY and ALIZA LEWKOWICZ, who fill me up with love every single day. I love you more than words can say.

To my grandchildren, SHALOM YISRAEL, ILAN ASHER, EMUNAH CHAYA, SHIFRA SHEFA-BRACHA & BEN-TZION NADEL, and ESTI, BATSHEVA, NOSSON TZVI & MOSHE SIMCHA LEWKOWICZ, who I love every inch of both inside and out.

To the rest of my FAMILY, for listening to my ideas about this book for a long time. Your love and patience is always appreciated. A special shout out to my sister and niece, SHARI and HEATHER BRODSKY, for their opinions and guidance; and to my brother-in-law, MICHAEL DETZKY, for his wealth of advice.

To my best friend, IRIS ROTH, for your constant support in everything that I do or try to do. You are the best friend anyone could ever have and I love you as a sister. I, also, thank your husband, LENNY, who welcomed me as family when you got married.

To my friend, PHYLLIS BLACKMAN, for being a committed friend who always gives the best advice.

And finally, to my co-author, HOPE STANGER, who enhanced my original concept for this book and equally contributed to the completion of it. Together, we have accomplished our goal of helping Jewish women be successful in losing weight, feeling great and looking great.

ABOVE ALL, I am grateful to HASHEM, the ultimate source of all our blessings.

THANK YOU FROM HOPE

I am grateful to G-d for every single moment of my life that led up to this book being brought into the world.

Thank you to my co-author, **GLORIA DAVIDSON**, for your collaboration on the birth of our book and its growth from a seed into a garden – May it bring you much nachas.

I want to express deep Gratitude to friends who supported me in all different ways to help this book come to life:

IDELE MOSKOWITZ: You have believed in me from the start and held me accountable to all of my book writing. Thank you for your inspirational check-in calls, lake-house retreat, guidance with the authors' conference and strong, loving friendship.

ELENOR LINDSAY: Thank you for being my Pioneer, and for offering me pillars of support and arms wide open through hours of phone calls. Thank you for also being my Book Angel and my dear friend.

ROSLYN TANNER EVANS: Thank you for your lifetime of friendship and your profound wisdom exactly when I needed it – and for talking and talking till everything made sense!

IRINA BRESLAV and **NICHOLAS LEPORE**: Thank you for batting around a multitude of concepts and ideas over fabulous raw food dinners together, and for being a collective sounding board of clarity and camaraderie.

ALLAN CHAPMAN: Thank you for your invaluable editing and insights for the authors' conference, and for your steadfast friendship – and lots of laughter through the process!

JULIA LATIMER: With immense gratitude for our shared vision and knowing that together, we would make it happen!

JOSHUA ROSENTHAL and the **INSTITUTE for INTEGRATIVE NUTRITION**®: Thank you for turning food on its right side!

My Dad, **ABRAHAM STANGER**: Thank you for instilling in me a love of words and language and the joy of sharing that together. May your memory be for a blessing. xoxo

My Mom, **CLAIRE STANGER**: Thank you for telling me I was a good writer from the time I was very young and giving me an amazing education. I love you. xoxo

It is my own journey that led me to this place of seeing how changing my beliefs could change the end result, and that changing how I spoke about my life could change those beliefs inside and make my dreams come true.

Thank you to all my guides and dear friends along the way.

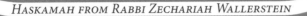

OHR NAAVA

women's · torah · center

founded in loving memory of Naava Katlowitz a"h

2201 East 23rd Street Brooklyn, NY 11229

718-OHR-NAAV(a) www.ohrnaava.com

I have read "Weigh Your Words and Throw Away your Scale!" in its entirety. This book, like its Authors, is full of sincerity, practical advice and better living for all Jewish women. Since it is targeted to help with the nutritional guidelines that they might be struggling with, which are not only limited to overeating or an eating disorder, I recommend that it be read carefully one section at a time with ample review for the best results.

This book is clearly the work of dedicated authors striving to help all Jewish women live a happier and healthier life style. May your goals in writing this book be a huge success not only to you but also to those that read and utilize the advice and strategies that you offer.

CONTENTS

INTRODUCTION

We decided to write this book for all the beautiful Jewish women of every background, shape and size who continually struggle with their weight. *WEIGH YOUR WORDS and THROW AWAY YOUR SCALE!*© is a 26-day **TOOL FOR WEIGHT LOSS** using the ABC's of the alphabet to help you lose weight and feel great through the power of positive speaking. It's to be used in **conjunction** with any weight loss plan or diet you choose and is designed as a support system or tool to enhance your ability to lose the weight and keep it off. With this book, you get to change your world by changing your words. As you make your way through the alphabet, you find words that are helpful during the process of losing weight as well as words to address the emotions that arise when you find yourself in difficult situations or with unhealthy food choices.

This book is an easy read and user-friendly tool, specifically designed for the busy lives of Jewish women and the many hats they wear. It's not going to weigh you down because it's designed to lighten you up. It's inspirational, motivational and easy to use; "as easy as ABC," because we believe that's what the process of weight loss should be. It's a small book that fits in your handbag and may just become your favorite new accessory! We designed it this way so you can easily carry and use it wherever you go to help override the desire to eat foods that do not support your weight loss goals. Each page has an alphabet letter with the *Word of the Day and Positive Intention* for you to speak out loud. Below that is a *Nutritional Action Step*, followed by a daily *Body Image Affirmation*, which you also get to speak aloud. As you are guided through the alphabet, you will also see a weekly *Reward System Reminder* – this is a time to give yourself an appreciation gift for believing in and following your goal of weight loss. It has been shown that we imprint new behaviors much more easily if we reward ourselves along the way. The back of the book contains a resources section entitled *Recipes and Tips*, which provides all the details you need to support the recommendations in the *Nutritional Action Steps*. Though this book goes along with whatever diet or weight-loss plan you decide upon or are already following, you are welcome to follow its nutritional guidelines as your primary weight-loss lifestyle as we have counseled many clients into weight-loss success with our methodology.

WEIGH YOUR WORDS and THROW AWAY YOUR SCALE! is a simple, clear and to-the-point book. It combines the power of positive speaking with behavioral actions, both known to produce lasting results and achievable goals. As a tool, its goal is to help support you in becoming a thinner and healthier woman and in appreciating all parts of yourself - acting as a supportive "friend" to accompany you on your weight-loss journey. We want you to speak it, believe it and finally own it, because we know when a woman owns her own greatness, change happens! You will find this book encouraging, uplifting and fun to follow as you successfully achieve your weight loss goals.

Weigh your words today so you can finally throw away your scale!

AND WE BEGIN WITH DAY 1...

The letter **A** is for **ACCOMPLISH.**

Say this in the morning and repeat it at least once during the day: "**I ACCOMPLISH** what I set out to do; I want to lose weight and **I DO!**"

Accomplishments come in small bites; not in big pieces. Every accomplishment, even a small one, is a big success in weight loss.

ACTION:

AVOCADOS make a delicious snack and are great for Shabbos salads and dips - or you can just slice one in half and eat it right out of its shell. When you're searching for something quick and easy to eat, this healthy fruit rich in nutrients is the perfect choice. Avocados reduce cravings for sweets and fried foods, help lower cholesterol levels and strengthen eye sight.

BODY IMAGE AFFIRMATION:

I take care of my health so I can **ALWAYS** serve Hashem and perform mitzvot.

DAY 2

The letter **B** is for **BELIEVE**.

Say this in the morning and repeat it at least once during the day: "I lose weight because **I BELIEVE IN MYSELF!** I'm confident and lose the weight I want to lose!"

When you think it you believe it, and when you speak it you make it real. Keep repeating this intention and notice how you feel.

ACTION:

BEETS are bold and help balance your blood sugar level and lift your cravings. They can be eaten raw or cooked. Always leave the skin on to get all your phytochemicals and antioxidants. Include beets and other root vegetables in your diet 3 times a week (see back of book for list of root veggies).

BODY IMAGE AFFIRMATION:

I keep my **BODY** healthy so I can better follow Hashem's wisdom and guidance.

DAY 3

The letter C is for CAPABLE.

Say this in the morning and repeat it at least once during the day: "**I AM CAPABLE** of changing the way that I eat; **I AM CAPABLE** of making healthy choices and changes!"

It's never black or white with weight loss. Look for the shades of grey in small changes. Make one small change today and it will be one large change from how you ate yesterday.

ACTION:

CANTALOUPE and other melons take only 15 minutes to digest so you should eat them early in the day before starting other foods. Packed with nutrients, they easily fill you up and help with weight loss. Keep them separate from protein and carbs to eliminate bloating. They can be chunked up, eaten whole or made into soups. Melons protect your heart, maintain your metabolism and help control blood pressure.

BODY IMAGE AFFIRMATION:

Hashem, please give me the **CHIZUK** (strength) to stay on my path of healthy weight loss.

DAY 4

The letter **D** is for **DETERMINED**.

Say this in the morning and repeat it at least once during the day: **"I AM DETERMINED** to lose weight and **I DO!** I have a strong and positive determination for losing weight!"

Keep going even if you take one step forward and two steps back because your determination will get you there. Each step is significant; the more determined you are, the more easily you will make lasting changes and meet your weight-loss goals.

ACTION:

VITAMIN D: Get out of your food rut and away from the refrigerator by going outside for a few minutes of sunshine, even in winter. Connecting with the sun elevates mood and supports weight-loss. Notice how much better you feel when you walk or even just stand under the sun for a few minutes a day. Include a vitamin D-rich food like salmon (see back of book for vitamin D foods).

BODY IMAGE AFFIRMATION:

I **DECIDE** to speak about myself as Hashem wants me to speak; with kindness.

DAY 5

The letter **E** is for EXERCISE.

Say this in the morning and repeat it at least once during the day: "I **EXERCISE** at every opportunity; I feel **GREAT** when I exercise!"

Weight loss and exercise go hand-in-hand. Here are some suggestions to bring in exercise wherever you are: Walk around when talking on the phone; if you are sitting on the couch, raise your arms, then make small and large circles in the air and do some leg lifts; when driving to the store, park a bit away so you have to walk. Include a few minutes of cardio-building and a few minutes of muscle-strengthening each day. Tip: Having a buddy to exercise with makes it more fun.

ACTION:

Add **ENERGY** into your diet with energy drinks by juicing once a day. Juicing is the way to get all your fruit and vegetable vitamins in a tall glass. It fills you with calcium, iron, potassium, and so much more. It also satisfies hunger, especially if you juice your favorites. Children love it, too (see back of book for fresh juice recipes). Juicing can be added in both as a meal or snack.

BODY IMAGE AFFIRMATION:

I **ELEVATE** my health by treating my body well.

DAY 6

The letter **F** is for **FOCUS**.

Say this in the morning and repeat it at least once during the day: **I FOCUS** on what I want in my life; **I FOCUS** on losing weight!"

Eat healthy and cut back on foods that are high in calories and fat. Focus on your portion control – you may want to consider eating more meals with smaller portions rather than fewer meals with larger portions.

ACTION:

FRESH FRUITS AND VEGETABLES support your body with far more vitamins, minerals, oxygen and energy than canned or frozen. It's the bright colors that make a difference. Eat tomatoes to help your heart and build your blood; have some yellow or orange peppers, golden beets or yellow squash to reduce inflammation; add purple cabbage to your salad to protect your nervous system. Each color helps us thrive so bring on the pineapple, blueberries and cherries!

BODY IMAGE AFFIRMATION:

I **FIND** time each day to thank Hashem for all he has given me.

DAY 7

The letter G is for GOAL.

Say this in the morning and repeat it at least once during the day: "**MY GOAL** is to lose weight and **KEEP IT OFF!**"

Make your weight-loss goals realistic so you never become frustrated. Decide upon a reasonable amount of weight loss that you know you can achieve and stick with your goal. "Don't put off till tomorrow what you can do today."

ACTION:

GO TO THE MARKET IN ADVANCE so you are never caught without. Always have healthy choices nearby. Even if your day goes differently than anticipated, you'll have something with you to eat. When planning your week think of meals, snacks and foods you can reach for when you're hungry.

BODY IMAGE AFFIRMATION:

I am filled with **GRATITUDE** to Hashem for every single day.

REWARD SYSTEM REMINDER:

You've completed your first week – now choose one way to reward yourself for this accomplishment. There is no size or category to the reward. It can be a present, small or large, an adventure you've been longing to take or anything that is completely just for you to receive. It can be as simple as taking a long nap or a walk in nature. The only requirement is to follow through on the reward, no matter what!

DAY 8

The letter H is for HEALTHY.

Say this in the morning and repeat it at least once during the day: "I know that I'm a **HEALTHIER PERSON** when I keep my body in shape. I choose to be **HEALTHY!**"

It's best to only keep foods in the house that support your weight-loss goals. Surround yourself with foods that nourish your body and help you lose weight. Let go of old temptations and replace them with new ones. Make sure you have plenty of healthy foods that you love.

ACTION:

HONOR YOUR HUNGER: When you're hungry, eat; don't wait to feed everyone else. Have some quick snacks nearby if it's not yet your mealtime – just enough healthy food to quiet your hunger and keep you focused on weight loss (see back of book for snack suggestions).

BODY IMAGE AFFIRMATION:

HASHEM is my guide and helps me keep my body strong.

DAY 9

The letter I is for I.

Say this in the morning and repeat it at least once during the day: "**I** lose weight for **ME** – to feel and look great!"

Lose weight for yourself – not for your spouse, mother, father, child/children, siblings or friend, because when you do it for yourself you really make it happen and it lasts!

ACTION:

INVESTIGATE YOUR BODY SIGNALS: Are you really hungry or just anxious, tired, lonely or overworked? Our relationship with food is a metaphor for so many other feelings, so take a breath and ask your body, "Is this hunger or something else?" Once you know, choose another activity for half an hour and see if it breaks the cycle.

BODY IMAGE AFFIRMATION:

Only Hashem in **HIS INFINITE** wisdom is able to give me exactly what I need to reach my potential.

DAY 10

The letter **J** is for JEWEL.

Say this in the morning and repeat it at least once during the day: "I am as **PRECIOUS** as a **JEWEL** and I sparkle more and more as I lose weight!"

Jewels are valued and treasured and so are you. Treat yourself with the care you give to your special gems because you are just as important. Lose the weight you want to lose to sparkle more and more each day.

ACTION:

JUMPSTART YOUR DAY WITH LEMON WATER: Drinking a tall glass of room temperature water (at least 16 oz.) with half of a fresh lemon squeezed in each morning cleans your liver of all the food it's had to process the day before. A good tip is to prepare it the night before and keep it on your nightstand. Drink your lemon water before you eat or drink anything else and you'll notice a difference in your day because it promotes energy and weight loss.

BODY IMAGE AFFIRMATION:

Today, I am happy to eat **JUST** what I need.

DAY 11

The letter K is for KICK OFF.

Say this in the morning and repeat it at least once during the day: "**I KICK OFF** my day with the positive belief that I can lose the weight I want to lose!"

Starting each day with positive thoughts and words helps you attain your weight-loss goals, so speak positive intentions every day.

ACTION:

KALE! is meant to be eaten regularly along with as many other leafy greens as possible. It's this category of vegetable that really helps you detoxify, lose weight, build your immune system and feel great! Leafies are also loaded with calcium (much more digestible calcium than dairy), potassium, vitamin E, iron, B vitamins, Omega 3's and protein. Add kale to your salad, sauté it or make kale chips for the whole family (see back of book for leafy greens recipes).

BODY IMAGE AFFIRMATION:

I am as **KIND** to myself as I am to others.

DAY 12

The letter L is for LOVE.

Say this in the morning and repeat it at least once during the day: "**I LOVE ME** and want to be healthy and happy!"

Love feels great – whether giving or receiving it. When you love yourself, you can love others so much more.

ACTION:

LISTEN TO YOUR BODY - LEARN WHAT FOODS HELP YOU FEEL GREAT: Check in with your body immediately after eating and later in your day. Ask yourself: Is there any change in my mood after eating (happy, sad, anxious)? How is my energy (tired, low, off-the-charts energized)? Any other feelings? Notice if there is a pattern and reduce the foods that lower your mood. If you like, start a "Food-Mood" journal to see it in writing.

BODY IMAGE AFFIRMATION:

I **LOOK** to Hashem to give me both mental and physical strength on my weight-loss journey.

DAY 13

The letter **M** is for **MYSELF**.

Say this in the morning and repeat it at least once during the day: "**I BELIEVE in MYSELF** and the healthy choices and changes I make with food!"

When you change one thing, you change more than you can imagine. Letting go of old habits and patterns happens one change at a time and all for the better.

ACTION:

MAKE EVERY MEAL COUNT: Each food we eat has the potential to make us feel better. Choose foods that give you energy for hours and boost your body with health. If you're eating a "white" (white flour, sugar or dairy), add in a "green" to alkalize your blood. On a Yom Tov, balance traditional foods by starting your day with a smoothie or healthy juice. Have a fresh green vegetable with your meat and make your meat the smaller part of your meal.

BODY IMAGE AFFIRMATION:

I MOTIVATE myself more and more each day to lose weight!

DAY 14

The letter **N** is for **NUTRITIOUS**.

Say this in the morning and repeat it at least once during the day: **I EAT NUTRITIOUS FOODS EVERY DAY** so I can be healthy, fit and lose weight!"

Your efforts with making good choices by eating healthy will pay off more and more. You will be able to do things you have been putting off, never did before, haven't been able to do for a long time or never would have considered doing at all. What you've dreamed of doing you will now start to do, feeling lighter with the food choices you have made.

ACTION:

NEVER SKIP A MEAL: Contrary to the philosophy behind all those years of yo-yo dieting, the best thing to do when eating more or different than normal is to go right back to your regular schedule. If you are still full from too much food, lighten up on the meal portion. When we skip, we send mixed messages to our bodies that backfire in the weight-loss process and trigger unhealthy diet habits. Stay with your plan and you'll be right back on track to weight loss.

BODY IMAGE AFFIRMATION:

Each day is a brand **NEW** moment in time to take care of my body and my health.

REWARD SYSTEM REMINDER

DAY 15

The letter O is for OPPORTUNITY.

Say this in the morning and repeat it at least once during the day: "**I CREATE OPPORTUNITIES** to eat healthy and lose weight!"

Opportunities come in abundance, so pause for a moment, then think about your best choice for weight-loss. Ask yourself what new opportunity you can create to help you succeed and go for it!

ACTION:

ORGANIZE YOUR FRIDGE AND CABINETS: It's great to have the right food choices around us but what if we can't find them? The answer is that the simpler we make our lives; the easier it is to meet our goals. Get rid of the foods that you no longer eat and fill your fridge and cabinets with your new, healthy energy foods. Put some reachable bowls of fruits, veggies and healthy choices front and center. Make sure you have plenty of delicious foods to choose from and don't skimp!

BODY IMAGE AFFIRMATION:

I **OPEN** myself up to new, healthier and better ways of eating every day.

DAY 16

The letter **P** is for **PERSON**.

Say this in the morning and repeat it at least once during the day: "I get an award for **PERSON OF THE YEAR** for my achievements in losing weight!"

Feel proud of what you've accomplished so far and be inspired to keep going! Look in the mirror and smile (really do this).

Action:

PREPARE FOR EACH DAY THE DAY BEFORE: When we set ourselves up for success, it easily comes our way. Make an action plan for your food and make sure you've got the foods you need. If you know you'll be busy or out, prepare foods that are easy to carry and eat. If you're going to be out for most of the day, bring a small cooler pack along. Always be prepared.

Body Image Affirmation:

I **PRAY** to Hashem and thank Him for his love and looking out for my good.

DAY 17

The letter Q is for QUEEN.

Say this in the morning and repeat it at least once during the day: "**I AM A QUEEN** because a **QUEEN** has the power to change things and make things happen!"

IT'S YOUR TIME TO BE A QUEEN! In the game of chess, the queen is the most powerful piece because she can move in any direction. Be a queen and move in the direction of weight loss.

ACTION:

Take a **QUANTUM LEAP** into health! Choose foods that leave you feeling light, powerful and focused; foods for your brain, body and weight loss. Eat just the right amount so you are clear and thriving with energy (see back of book for list of brain-boosting foods).

BODY IMAGE AFFIRMATION:

I take **QUIET** time to connect with each meal I eat.

DAY 18

The letter **R** is for **REAL**.

Say this in the morning and repeat it at least once during the day: **"I'M KEEPING IT REAL** with my food choices today!"

Exercise and keep eating healthy; the more you do it, the more you'll want to! The positive results you'll see and feel will bring you long-lasting satisfaction every single day.

ACTION:

REST WHEN YOU ARE TIRED: Lack of sleep so often triggers hunger in the form of cravings. We try to make up with food what we are missing with rest and reach for the wrong foods instead. Get clear on bed time and let go of sending that last email or text. Energy and focus promote weight loss.

BODY IMAGE AFFIRMATION:

When I **RISE** in the morning, I express gratitude to Hashem for graciously restoring my soul to me so that I may worship Him anew.

DAY 19

The letter **S** is for **SUCCESS!**

Say this in the morning and repeat it at least once during the day: I am **SUCCEEDING** with my goal for losing weight – I am a **WEIGHT-LOSS SUCCESS!**"

Stay inspired and empowered with believing that you have the power to succeed and you will!

ACTION:

IT'S TIME FOR SMOOTHIES! We can pack so many vitamins and nutrients into a blended drink, and drinking smoothies is one of our favorite weight-loss tips. When we let go of chewing for one meal, our body gets to detoxify and digest; it doesn't have to work so hard and it promotes weight loss. Our favorite is a raw cacao smoothie – it's a chocolate drink that clients say is the most satisfying and delicious treat (see cacao smoothie and other smoothie recipes in back).

BODY IMAGE AFFIRMATION:

I **SHOWER** myself with healthy foods, daily exercise, loving thoughts and prayer.

DAY 20

The letter **T** is for **TRANSFORMATION**.

Say this in the morning and repeat it at least once during the day: "I **TRANSFORM** the way I think about food and the way I eat food – I **TRANSFORM** my relationship with food!"

Any transformation that takes place is a process and to accomplish it is victorious. Be proud of the changes you are making inside and out.

Action:

TASTE EVERY BITE WITH ALL OF YOUR SENSES and TAKE YOUR TIME: Eating quickly is something many of us struggle with and it adds on pounds. Before we've actually even tasted the first bite, we're onto the next. Slow down and start to experience your food. See what happens when you notice all the taste sensations. Take a bite, chew it slowly and completely until liquefied and swallow. Then put your fork back in.

Body Image Affirmation:

TESHUVA, TEFILLAH and TZEDAKAH help me meet my weight-loss goals.

DAY 21

The letter **U** is for **UNDERSTAND**.

Say this in the morning and repeat it at least once during the day: **"I UNDERSTAND** the significance of losing weight to make me **FEEL** and **LOOK GREAT - I REALLY UNDERSTAND."**

You are aware of the importance and benefits of weight loss and are learning much about food, health and your body. The more you learn, the more you understand and the more you can do. Awareness and understanding are the keys to action.

ACTION:

UNVEIL ONE NEW RECIPE A WEEK: We know for sure that "getting your hands in the food" connects you more closely to your body and weight-loss goals. Find recipes that contain some of your favorite foods made healthy, and buy the ingredients in advance. Cooking is an amazing act of self-care. We are not just eating blindly; we're developing a relationship with our food.

BODY IMAGE AFFIRMATION:

I **FEEL UPLIFTED** when I see my progress with weight loss.

REWARD SYSTEM REMINDER

DAY 22

The letter V is for VOCALIZE.

Say this in the morning and repeat it at least once during the day: **"I VOCALIZE MY POSITIVE INTENTION DAILY** because I know when I say it I lose the weight and keep it off!"

You are doing great with following all parts of this book – the positive intention, nutritional action step and body image affirmation. Keep saying your Positive Intention out loud, because when you say it, you make it happen.

ACTION:

VISUALIZE YOURSELF THIN! Experiencing ourselves as if who we want to be is already so is a powerful and effective way to reach our desired goal. The more we see it, think it, smell it, taste it, touch it and believe it, the more we become the thin woman we know we can be. Each morning, take sixty seconds to imagine yourself the way you want to look. Picture yourself choosing an outfit, getting dressed and walking out the door thin. Really see yourself as the person you know is inside of you. Feel who she is when she has met her goals.

BODY IMAGE AFFIRMATION:

I am **VERY** loved by Hashem. Treating myself with love is a direct reflection of Hashem's love.

DAY 23

The letter W is for WELCOME.

Say this in the morning and repeat it at least once during the day: "**I WELCOME A WORLD** of **HEALTHY EATING** on my weight-loss journey!

Because you're almost at the end of our book, you've already learned and implemented so much to support you in losing weight and feeling great. Continue with your welcome world of weight loss. Stay positive and do what you're doing.

ACTION:

WAIT BEFORE GIVING INTO A CRAVING – CHANGE YOUR THOUGHT AND LOCATION: If you're feeling shaky, hungry, tired, anxious or just having a really big craving, pause, and try this: Think about something completely different. Choose a thought about a positive and happy event, person or moment in your life. At the same time, move yourself to another location – if you are in the living room, go to another room; if you're out in a store, move to a different department. This simple act rewires the brain and stops the craving.

BODY IMAGE AFFIRMATION:

Hashem, I ask that you continue to guide me on my **WEIGHT-LOSS** journey.

DAY 24

The letter X is for **eXtra**.

Say this in the morning and repeat it at least once during the day: "**I LOSE** all the **eXtra** weight I want to lose and continue on my path to meet my weight-loss goals!"

You are losing weight because you can! See how wonderful and uplifted you feel becoming the lighter you. Stay encouraged, be inspired and keep on going!

ACTION:

I AM ON THE X-AXIS – I STAY ON COURSE. It's simple: Today, just go from left to right in a straight line with your food, exercise and thoughts. Don't think too hard; just follow this path to success.

BODY IMAGE AFFIRMATION:

I feel **eXceptional** with my devotion to my health and weight loss!

DAY 25

The letter Y is for YES!

Say this in the morning and repeat it at least once during the day: "**YES**, I'm doing it – **EATING HEALTHY** and **LOSING WEIGHT** – **YES, I AM!**"

Feel great about what you've accomplished; you have just one more letter to go to complete this book! Focus on how good you feel and look with the weight you've lost so far, and how staying positive keeps you inspired and believing in yourself. Just keep **SAYING YES!**

ACTION:

YOU – TODAY IS ALL ABOUT YOU AND YOU GET TO WEIGH YOUR WORDS! It's Day 25, and you're in the swing of it, so here's your chance to personalize our method. Make up your own, "*Positive Intention, Nutritional Action Step* and *Body Image Affirmation*," using any letter that you like. You get to decide today. Just follow our lead and insert your own sentences. See the very back of our book for the "*Weigh Your Words by You*" pages, where you can add your own words. If you're having so much fun doing this and want to create more, we've left you extra space to invent new ideas for weight-loss success.

BODY IMAGE AFFIRMATION:

I lose weight and feel great with **YOUR** guidance, Hashem. Thank you for helping me to do this.

DAY 26

The letter Z is for ZEST!

Say this in the morning and repeat it at least once during the day: **"I HAVE A ZEST FOR LOSING WEIGHT and a ZEST FOR LIFE!"**

Your zest has paid off! All your enthusiasm to lose weight – to feel and look great – has brought you here; to the end of the alphabet and the end of our 26-day plan. People who have zest complete things with enthusiasm and motivation and perform them wholeheartedly. You are this person! Continue to keep this positive trait of **ZEST** you exude and always approach life with energy and excitement.

ACTION:

STAY IN YOUR ZONE: Using the *Weigh Your Words* alphabet daily keeps you exactly where you want to be; in the zone of losing weight and feeling great. Congratulate yourself on reaching the final letter! You should keep this book by your side for daily guidance and inspiration, and feel free to reread it at anytime. It's here to support you all day long; every single day, like a friend by your side.

BODY IMAGE AFFIRMATION:

I thank you Hashem, a **ZILLION** times, for helping me to care for my body, choose my food wisely and meet my weight-loss goals!

FINAL REWARD SYSTEM REMINDER

Mazel Tov!

You made it through the alphabet! Give yourself something large enough to acknowledge all of your hard work and dedication. You have stuck to your commitment and that's **HUGE!**

AUTHOR'S NOTE

Weigh Your Words and Throw Away Your Scale! is designed to be a friend for life - you can keep it by your side and read it as many times as you like to stay on track, whether you've met your weight-loss goals or are still in the process. Once you've lost all the weight and want to keep eating in the zone of health, we suggest you continue to say our *Positive Intentions* to remind you to you feel great about yourself every day. Our desire for you is that you always use your words instead of the scale!

We wish you much success!
Gloria and Hope

RECIPES AND TIPS

All of our recipes are geared for energy and weight loss and detail the *Nutritional Action Step* recommendations.

Our food categories are listed in alphabetical order so the recipes are easy to find.

Food category #1

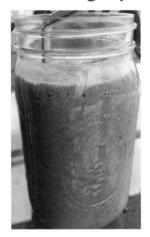

JUICES

Juices are food for life! When we juice a vegetable or fruit, we eliminate its fiber and make it more easily digestible. It detoxifies our body for weight loss and health and strengthens our immune system. We are unable to eat the amount of fruits and vegetables in a day that can accomplish what one tall glass of juice does.

We recommend having 16-32 oz. of juice per day. Keep all skins on your vegetables and just give them a rinse or scrub with a brush. Drink your juice within a few minutes of preparing it to get all the nutrients. You'll need a juicer and your fruits and vegetables, and you're all set to go. Lots of places sell fresh juices, too. We recommend buying organic to eliminate pesticides.

Here is our favorite green juice and our favorite fruit juice:

ALL GREEN JUICE WITH APPLE AND GINGER

(the best juice for weight loss, immune building and detoxification)

INGREDIENTS:

10 leafy green leaves, using any mix of leafy greens (see leafy greens' list)

1 green apple

1 bunch of parsley, cilantro or a mix of both

2 stalks of celery

1 cucumber

¼ fresh lemon

½ inch – 1 inch fresh ginger root

Option: 2 Carrots

DIRECTIONS:

Alternate vegetables and apple back and forth, putting some of each type down the juice shoot with its plunger until all the juice is extracted.

Pour the juicing pitcher juice into a tall glass and squeeze in lemon.

Drink within 15 minutes.

CANTELOUPE COOLER

INGREDIENTS:

1 cantaloupe

1 orange

1 box strawberries

1 cucumber

3 leaves of Swiss chard

¼ fresh lemon

DIRECTIONS:

Alternate fruit and vegetables back and forth, putting some of each type down the juice shoot with its plunger until all the juice is extracted.

Pour the juicing pitcher juice into a tall glass and squeeze in lemon.

Drink within 15 minutes.

Food category #2

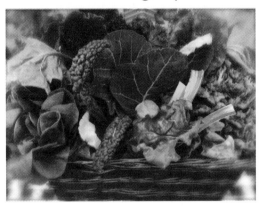

LEAFY GREENS

The most important category of vegetables, leafy greens supply us with our life force energy. They are packed with vitamins, minerals and phytonutrients. They bring oxygen to all of our cells and strengthen our immune system, lowering our risk of disease. They are also packed with protein!

Here are the most popular leafy greens:

Kale, Swiss Chard, Collard Greens, Spinach, Arugula, Bok Choy and Watercress

KALE APPLE SALAD

Here's a wonderful and easy way to eat kale – no need to even cook!

INGREDIENTS:

1 bunch of kale	2 swirls extra virgin olive oil
1 large apple	1 teaspoon Dijon mustard
1 ripe avocado	1 teaspoon raw honey
1 swirl apple cider vinegar	Raw, unsalted sunflower seeds

DIRECTIONS:

Tear the leaves away from the stems of the kale and tear them up. Chop up some of the stems and toss both into a large bowl. Add the avocado in pieces. Swirl apple cider vinegar once around. Swirl olive oil twice around. Add mustard and honey.

Using your hands, knead the kale, avocado and dressing for a full 1-2 minutes, as if you are kneading bread.

Add in the sunflower seeds and toss. We get lots of compliments on this salad when serving it to guests. It stays well for a number of days in the fridge.

KALE CHIPS

Are you craving something crunchy, salty and satisfying that won't add weight to your body?

INGREDIENTS:

1 large bunch of kale   Sea salt

Olive oil or coconut oil

DIRECTIONS:

Tear leaves away from stems and into large pieces.

Put into bowl and toss with oil and sea salt to taste.

Lay on trays or cookie sheets (grease with oil).

Bake at 350 degrees until crispy.

Food category #3

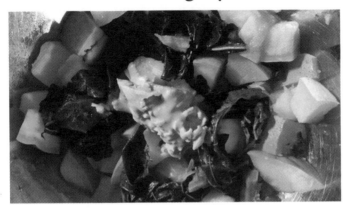

ROOT VEGETABLES

These incredible vegetables that grow low into the ground are powerful healing tools. On the emotional end, they help us stay calm. They are great for stress and anxiety. On the physical end, they help stabilize blood sugar levels and reduce cravings for sweets.

Here is a list of some root veggies:

Beets, Carrots, Sweet Potato, Onion, Turnip, Rutabaga, Parsnip and Radish

Include all squashes in this family, too – **Zucchini, Yellow Squash, Acorn Squash and Butternut Squash**

BEETS: Strengthen the heart, improve circulation, build red blood cells and reduce cravings for junk food.

Here is a wonderful root vegetable recipe from Hope's alma mater, the *Institute for Integrative Nutrition®*:

SWEET SENSATION

Almost everyone craves sweets. Rather than depending on processed sugar to satisfy cravings, add naturally sweet foods to your daily diet to satisfy your sweet tooth.

Sweet vegetables soothe the internal organs of the body and energize the mind. And because many of these vegetables are root vegetables, they help to balance out the spaciness people often feel after eating other kinds of sweet foods. Adding in sweet vegetables helps to crowd out less healthy foods in the diet.

INGREDIENTS:

Use a few of the root vegetables mentioned above

Water for cooking

DIRECTIONS:

Chop the hardest vegetables, like carrots and beets, into smaller pieces.

Softer vegetables, like onions can be cut into larger chunks. Use a medium-sized pot and add enough water to barely cover the vegetables. You may want to check the water level while cooking and add more water if needed. Remember, vegetables on the bottom will get cooked more than the ones on the top. Cook until desired softness. The softer the vegetables get, the sweeter they become.

When the vegetables are cooked to your satisfaction, empty the ingredients into a large bowl, flavor as desired and eat. The leftover cooking water makes a delicious sweet sauce and is a healing, soothing tonic to drink by itself.

STEAMED BUTTERNUT SQUASH WITH TAHINI AND TAMARI

INGREDIENTS:

½ Butternut Squash, with skin on

Tamari – to taste (gluten-free soy sauce made by San-J; optional for those regulating salt intake)

Tahini – to taste

2 tablespoons coconut oil

Splash of olive oil

Sea salt – to taste

Herbs and spices of choice

DIRECTIONS:

In a steamer pot, put 2 inches of water and place the steamer on top.

With a sharp knife, first cut the squash in half, removing and saving any seeds. Refrigerate half the squash. Continue by slicing the remaining squash into thick rounds and then cutting it into medium-sized chunks. Remove all remaining seeds, save and place the pieces of squash in the steamer.

Bring the water to a boil; cover pot and continue boiling (you can adjust to a slightly-lower boiling temp) till squash is tender when you insert a fork.

Remove and place in bowl.

Splash some tamari over the squash and drizzle the tahini.

You can put the seeds in a bowl and toss with coconut oil, a little olive oil, sea salt and any herbs and spices you like.

Spread the seeds out on parchment paper or a tray greased with coconut oil.

Bake at 350 degrees till crispy.

The seeds will keep in a container and are a great vitamin-rich snack.

Food Category #4

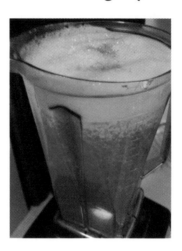

SMOOTHIES!

Smoothies are a delicious way to make a healthy shake filled with protein, vitamins, minerals and many more nutrients than we could ever chew in the same sitting. Unlike juices, they are packed with fiber and can also sustain you with energy for hours. If you want a boost in the morning, it's a simple way to include a power-packed breakfast. It's great as a snack or for other meals, too. Children absolutely love smoothies – they can choose the fruits and vegetables they like and help you with the blending.

You will need a high-speed, strong blender that can blend fruits and vegetables. We recommend drinking 24-32 oz. of smoothie at a time.

Here are our most favorite smoothie recipes:

RAW CACAO CHOCOLATE SMOOTHIE:

This drink will help you give up coffee, boost your energy and eliminate cravings. Our clients swear by it. Raw chocolate, known as cacao, contains iron, magnesium, calcium, potassium and antioxidants. It improves cell function. More importantly, it increases and balances your serotonin levels, helping you feel happy and content – it actually mimics the way you feel when you're in love! Cacao gives the brain a boost without caffeine; it has theobromine.

INGREDIENTS:

2 ½ cups chilled coconut water

1 frozen banana (take ripe bananas, peel them and put them whole in a freezer bag in the freezer – you can pull out one as needed)

1 scoop (coffee scooper) raw cacao powder (in vitamin/ supplement section of health food store)

3 tablespoons chia seeds (in vitamin/supplement section of health food store)

1 heaping tablespoon raw honey

Option: Add some fresh strawberries

DIRECTIONS:

Pour coconut water into blender. Break the frozen banana in two or three pieces and add to blender. Add all other ingredients. Cover and blend. You can drink right away or chill in the freezer for ten minutes.

WATERMELON, STRAWBERRY, LIME SMOOTHIE:

Watermelon is the most nutrient-dense fruit around and is our personal summer favorite. It is also 91.5% water for hydration.

INGREDIENTS:

1 large round slice of watermelon (1 inch thick)

10 strawberries

½ lime

DIRECTIONS:

Cut the watermelon meat off of the rind and put into the blender. Add the strawberries and lime and blend.
Enjoy!

KALE-BANANA-MANGO SMOOTHIE:

INGREDIENTS:

2 ½ cups coconut water

3 leaves kale

1 frozen banana

1 ripe mango

3 tablespoons chia seeds

1 tablespoon coconut oil

DIRECTIONS:

Starting with the coconut water, add all ingredients to blender. Break the frozen banana into pieces before adding. Peel the mango first, discarding the pit and adding the fruit. Tear the kale into smaller pieces and add.

Blend and serve!

SPINACH-AVOCADO SMOOTHIE SOUP:

Here's a dinner smoothie:

INGREDIENTS:

1 bunch spinach, rinsed well

1 avocado

1 red pepper

2 ½ cups almond milk

1 clove garlic

Cayenne pepper to taste (for spiciness)

Sea salt - to taste

Tamari - to taste

DIRECTIONS:

Rinse and add all ingredients into blender, starting with the almond milk. Blend till smooth.

Chill in refrigerator till cool and serve.

Food Category #5

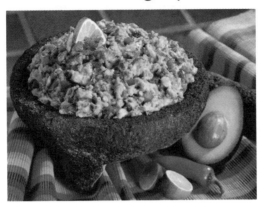

SNACKS

Our favorite snacks are also great at mealtime.

AVOCADOS

Avocados contain potassium (more than bananas!), vitamin K, folate, vitamin C and vitamins B5, B6 and E. They are loaded with fiber as well, and contain protein, carbohydrates and healthy fat. Guacamole is wonderful for lunch, dinner or a snack.

GUACAMOLE FOR 1:

INGREDIENTS:

1 ripe avocado	¼ fresh lemon
1 ripe tomato	Sea salt – to taste
½ onion	Cayenne pepper – to taste

DIRECTIONS:

Scoop avocado out of its shell and put into bowl. Chop up tomato and add in. Chop up onion and add in. Squeeze in lemon.

Start with ¼ teaspoon sea salt and add to taste.

Add in 1 or 2 shakes of cayenne, adding slowly to taste for heat and spiciness.

Mash with a fork, making the guacamole creamier but still keeping all the veggies chunky.

If you're making it for the family use 3 ripe avocados, two tomatoes and a whole onion. Squeeze ½ lemon, ½ teaspoon sea salt and season to taste.

BEANS

Beans are an excellent substitute for meat. They're the perfect balance of high protein, high carbs, high fiber and low fat. They are also loaded with calcium, magnesium, phosphorous, potassium and B vitamins, thiamin, iron and folate.

BEAN PATÉ

Here's a bean recipe – a great shot of plant-based protein that is easy to make on the run. Enjoy it as a snack or with your meal.

INGREDIENTS:

1 can of kidney or northern beans (preferably organic)

Olive oil

Sea salt – to taste

2 cloves fresh garlic

1-2 tablespoons tahini

Water

DIRECTIONS:

Rinse and drain the beans – then pour into a blender or food processor.

Add a couple of big splashes of olive oil, garlic, ¼ teaspoon sea salt and 1 tablespoon tahini.

Blend all ingredients. Check the flavor and add more salt and tahini as desired.

Helpful Hints:

Add the olive oil until you get the desired consistency when blending or processing – some people like it to look like hummus and others like a chunkier blend.

Add water to make it more blendable and thinner – just a little bit at a time.

Use as a spread or just eat with a spoon!

Food Category #6

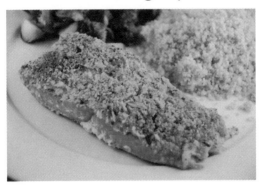

VITAMIN D is essential for bone and teeth health and can prevent osteoporosis and lift your mood.

VITAMIN D FOODS

Fatty Fish - Salmon, Tuna, Herring, Halibut, Trout, Sardines and Mackerel; Shitake Mushrooms; Eggs; Cod Liver Oil

SIMPLE SALMON:

Four ingredients turn your fish into a rich and scrumptious dish. The organic flaxseeds are high in Omega-3 fatty acids and make a perfect topping.

INGREDIENTS: (per individual salmon steak or fillet)

    1-2 tablespoons olive oil

    1 teaspoon Dijon mustard

    2 tablespoons coarsely ground flaxseeds

    ½ teaspoon raw honey

DIRECTIONS:

    In a glass, combine ingredients and mix. Spread over fish and bake at 350 degrees until cooked on the outside but still a little pink on the inside.

Food category #7

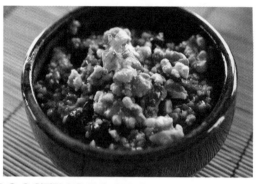

BRAIN-BOOSTING FOODS

Wild Alaskan Salmon, Broccoli, Cauliflower, Walnuts, Tomatoes, Celery, Blueberries, Coconut Oil, Pumpkin Seeds, Turmeric (spice) and Whole Grains (complex carbohydrates; healthy carbs!) - Quinoa, Millet, Kasha, Brown Rice, Barley and Oats

Whole grains are low in fat and calories and high in energy!

BRAIN-BOOSTING BREAKFAST: This delicious whole grain recipe will sustain you for hours, leaving you feeling full and energized.

INGREDIENTS:

½ cup steel cut oats

1 ½ cups of water

¼ cup coconut milk

1 handful of raw almonds

2 handfuls of raisins

DIRECTIONS:

Put water and grain in pot and bring to a boil, uncovered on stovetop.

Lower temperature to medium low; add in almonds and raisins and cover to cook.

Cook until the water is absorbed. Turn off burner. Add coconut milk without stirring and re-cover the pot, letting it sit for 5 minutes. Uncover and stir. Time to eat!

MUSHROOM & BARLEY SIDE DISH

INGREDIENTS:

½ cup pearled barley

1½ cups water

½ lb. mushrooms, sliced

½ onion, chopped

1 heaping tablespoon coconut oil

Olive oil – to taste

Sea salt – to taste

DIRECTIONS:

In a medium-sized skillet, heat 1 heaping tablespoon of coconut oil. Add in the mushrooms and onions and sauté. When veggies are cooked but not too soft, put them on a covered plate and set aside.

Put water and barley in a pot and bring to a boil uncovered on stovetop.

Lower temperature to medium-low, cover and cook until all water is absorbed. Turn off burner and let sit covered for 5 minutes. Uncover, add in mushrooms and stir. Drizzle with olive oil and add sea salt to taste.

To serve more people use 1 cup of barley, 2 ½ cups water, 1 lb. of mushrooms and 1 onion.

Food Category #8

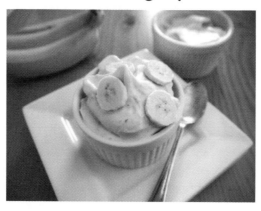

QUICK, SWEET AND HEALTHY!

Reach for these recipes when you want something sweet and comforting. They will satisfy a sugar craving and still help you continue to lose weight. You can eat them as dessert or for a snack.

BANANA ICE CREAM

INGREDIENTS:

1 frozen banana

¼ cup raisins

¼ cup shredded unsweetened coconut

DIRECTIONS:

Break banana into four pieces and put in food processor. Add remaining ingredients and process till creamy.

Note: For a whole family, use 1 banana per person and increase raisins and coconut.

CRUNCHY DATES

INGREDIENTS:

3 large dates   3 raw almonds or walnuts

DIRECTIONS:

Split open each date and remove its pit.

Insert an almond or walnut in place of the pit.

Walnuts are meatier; almonds are crunchier.

Enjoy!

These are some of our many recipes and recommendations for healthy food choices to lose weight and feel great. Use them to support your *Nutritional Action Steps* together with your *Positive Intention* and *Body Image Affirmation* for weight-loss success.

ABOUT THE AUTHORS

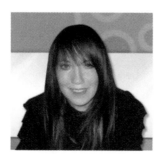

Gloria Davidson is an image consultant and a food and dating coach. She is also the inventor of Destination Wig - traveling wig stand. Gloria gives lectures and teaches classes about Image from Head to Toe and believes your style is a way to express who you are. As an observant Jewish woman, she always wants women to feel confident and gives them the knowledge to project their personal style because she knows every woman is unique. She helps single, married, divorced and widowed women discover the key to effortless image and identifies the ideal look for them. She has also helped her clients lose weight through the methodology outlined in this book resulting in increased self-confidence for dating, marriage, weight loss and business success. Through her company, *Number 1 Image*, Gloria focuses on single women by helping them create a dynamic dating profile and photo image to find their happily ever after. Gloria resides with her husband Mendy in Woodmere, New York. Together, their children and grandchildren live throughout New York, Michigan and Israel. To find out more about working with Gloria in an individualized counseling program please email her at Gloriaweighyourwords@gmail.com

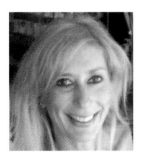

Hope Stanger is a trauma therapist, nutritional counselor and sought-after motivational speaker in practice for over fifteen years. She is an expert in the field of Transformational Nutrition. In her personal journey of weight loss, she went from weighing two hundred and twenty pounds to losing over eighty pounds. Seeing this in her own life inspired her to become a nutritional therapist and eventually bring the methodology outlined in this book to others. She has worked with hundreds of women, teaching them how to have joyful, peaceful and powerful relationships with their food, body and health. She is a graduate of the *Institute for Integrative Nutrition*. Hope developed a new model in therapy to heal trauma, relationships and eating disorders and is the founder of *Therapy Beyond Walls*, counseling individuals, couples and groups worldwide. She lives by the beach in Stamford, Connecticut. To find out more about working with Hope in an individualized counseling program please email her at Hope@weighyourwordsandthrowawayyourscale.com

"WEIGH YOUR WORDS BY YOU"

Positive Intention:

Action:

Body Image Affirmation:

Positive Intention:

Action:

Body Image Affirmation:

Positive Intention:

Action:

Body Image Affirmation:

THANK YOU TO OUR SPONSORS FOR BELIEVING IN OUR BOOK

GOURMET GLATT
With appreciation to Yoeli Steinberg, Chanie Friedman and Esther Schwartz

SIERRA TUCSON
With appreciation to Julia Latimer, Lisa Jane Vargas, Alison Broderick and Cheryl LaPlant

In memory of our mother,
HELEN NICHTER
who found beauty in every person
-Mark and Alvin

SPECIAL THANKS TO our publisher, Akiva Atwood, and the staff at Targum Press. Your guidance and patience with the creation and production of this book has been immeasurable, from inception to completion.

Where stories are shared and troubles unburdened

Where children are encouraged to be seen *and* heard

Where workday concerns shrink down to the size of a cholent bean

Where an empty chair is an eloquent invitation

Where milestones are marked with favorite foods and the simple gift of remembering

Where new friendships are nourished by warm smiles and hot chicken soup

Where "Bubby's Best-Ever Chocolate Cake" is garnished with the sweetest of memories

Where traditions are both preserved and created

Where laughter, love and a sense of belonging are always on the menu

Thank you for honoring us with *a place at your table*

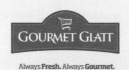
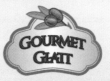

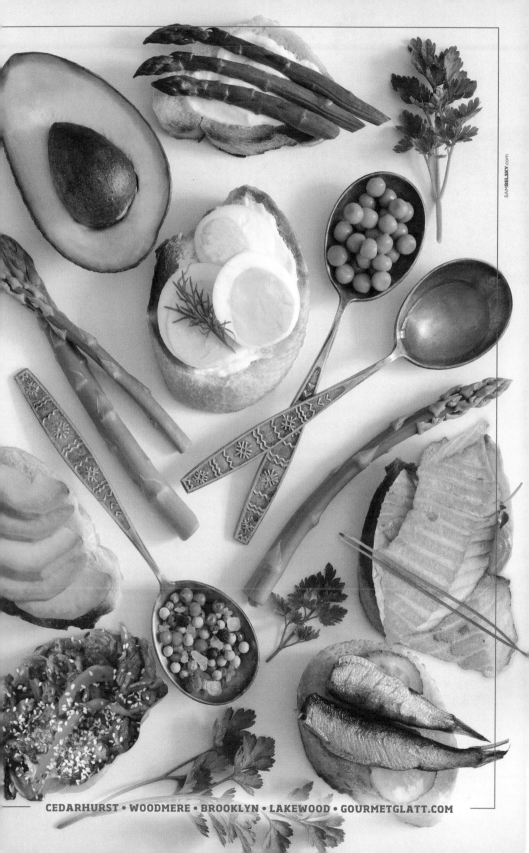

CEDARHURST • WOODMERE • BROOKLYN • LAKEWOOD • GOURMETGLATT.COM

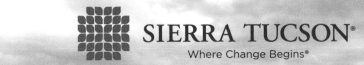

SIERRA TUCSON®
Where Change Begins®

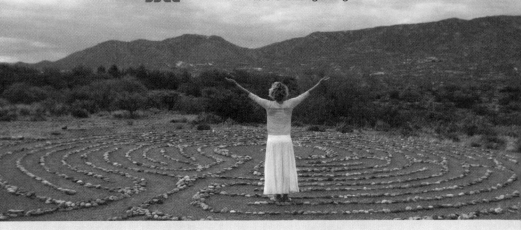

A Message from Our Sponsor

In an effort to raise awareness about the importance of cultural sensitivity in the behavioral health field, Sierra Tucson—a residential treatment center located in Tucson, Arizona—is partnering with authors Hope Stanger and Gloria Davidson to support the message of their book and the need for resources that are tailored for Jewish women. Our Cultural Sensitivity Program is designed to honor the values and beliefs of Jewish women through all levels of religious observance. For Orthodox women in treatment, we provide residents with glatt-kosher meals and food plans; respect laws of observance, including the Sabbath; recognize tzniut guidelines; and accommodate Jewish customs, traditions and lifestyle. Staff members receive cultural diversity training from a Sierra Tucson Cultural Sensitivity Liaison, allowing our multidisciplinary team of professionals to customize each woman's treatment plan according to her cultural needs.

Since 1983, Sierra Tucson has been an internationally renowned leader in comprehensive residential treatment, employing cutting-edge integrative therapies and evidence-based practices for behavioral and psychiatric disorders. Our longstanding legacy of clinical excellence and compassionate care has resulted in recovery for those struggling with eating disorders, trauma-related issues, substance use disorder, chronic pain, and mood and anxiety disorders. Situated on a serene 160-acre campus, Sierra Tucson offers a safe, supportive environment for those in need of hope and healing.

For more information about Sierra Tucson's Cultural Sensitivity Program for Jewish women, visit SierraTucson.com.